D0843249

TIGER LIVY

Erin Garcia and Betsy Miller
Illustrated by Ivreese Tong

To anyone who needs healing and
the beautiful people who help them.

One lovely spring day, Livy played and pounced with her friends.

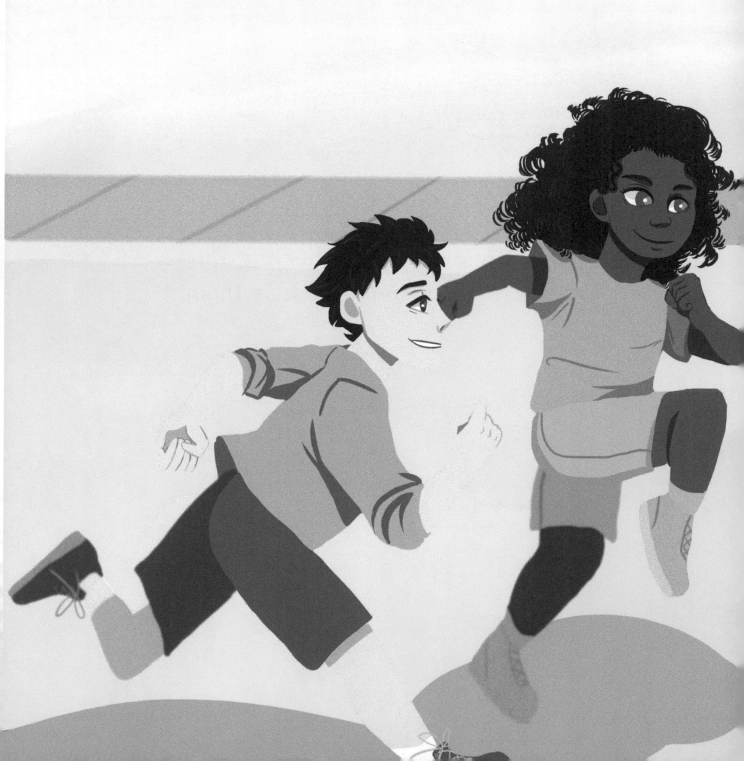

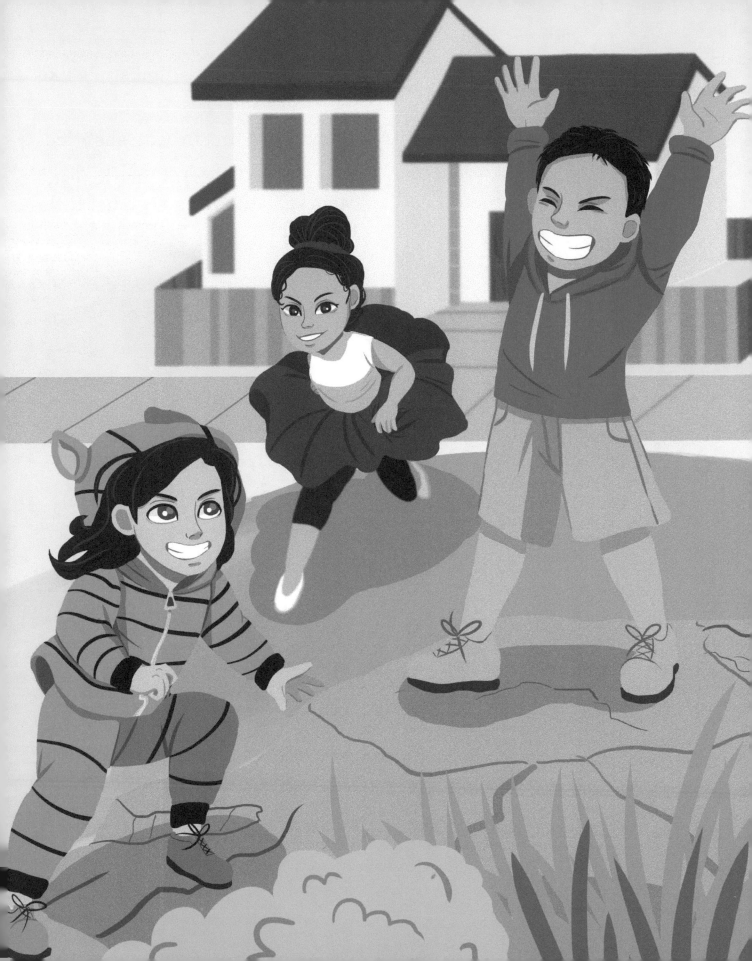

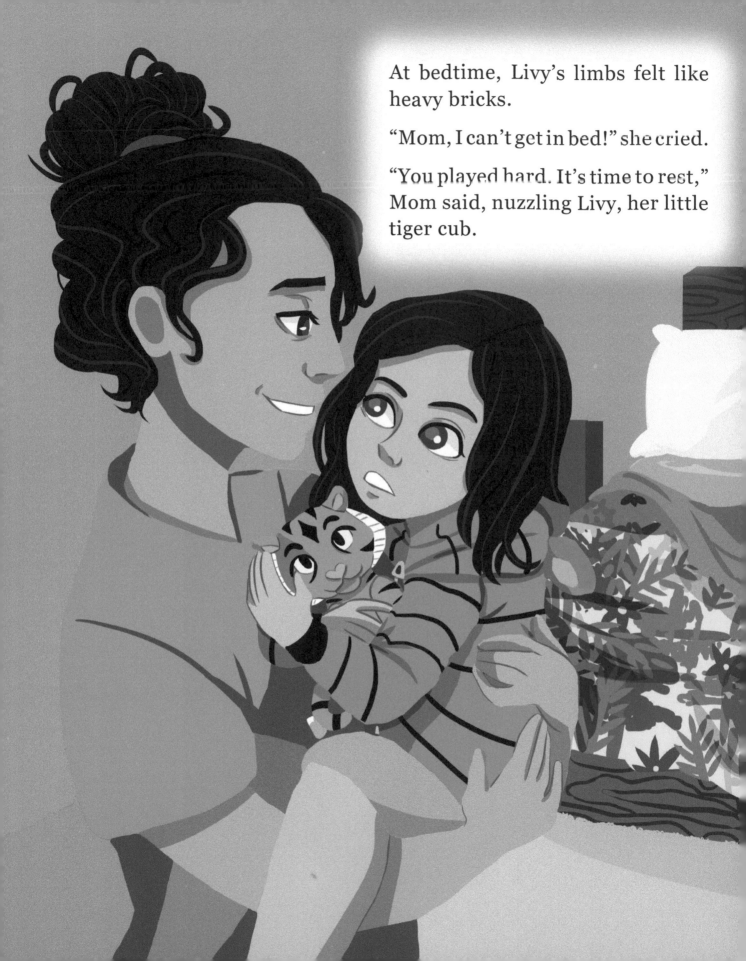

At bedtime, Livy's limbs felt like heavy bricks.

"Mom, I can't get in bed!" she cried.

"You played hard. It's time to rest," Mom said, nuzzling Livy, her little tiger cub.

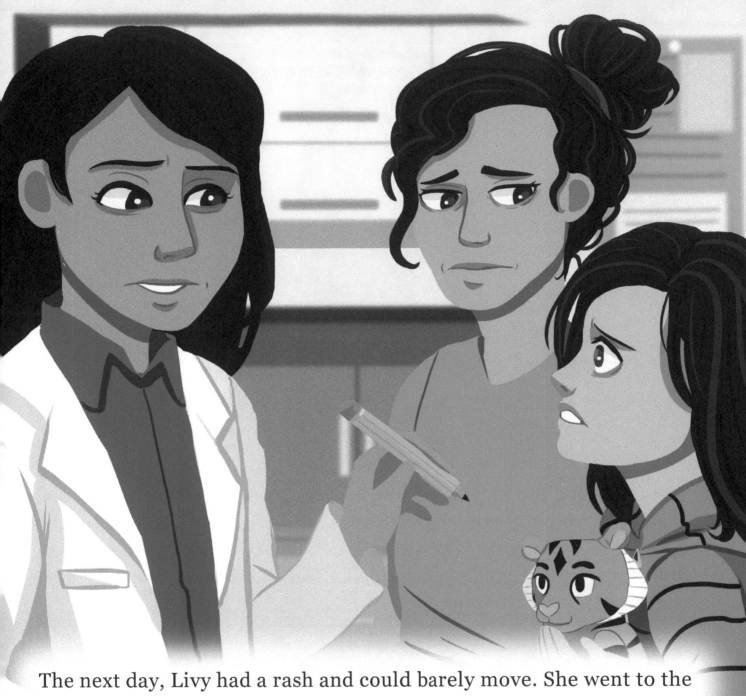

The next day, Livy had a rash and could barely move. She went to the doctor. "Did I play too much?" Livy asked.

"Oh no," the doctor replied. "You're sick and your body needs extra help to heal this kind of disease. We're not sure how long it will take. We do know you need strong medicine, healthy food, and rest."

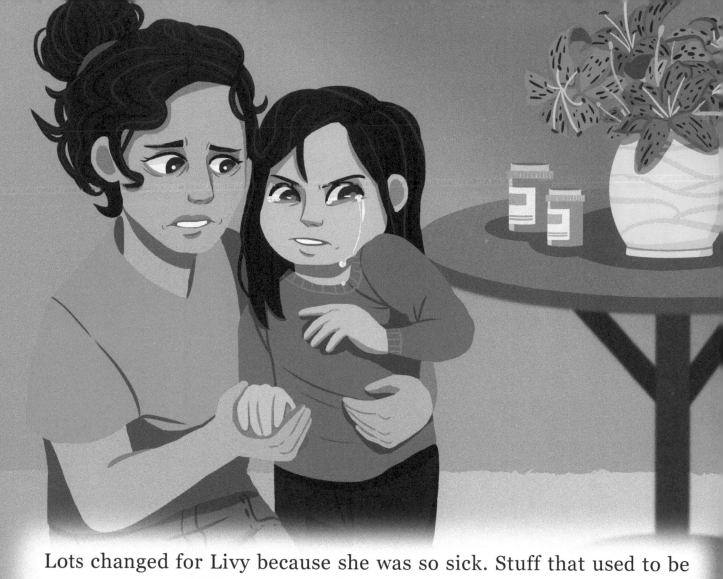

Lots changed for Livy because she was so sick. Stuff that used to be easy was now difficult. Little things made her cry. Mom held Livy close and explained, "The strong medicine is fighting your disease, but it also might make you suddenly feel sad or mad. We call this a side effect."

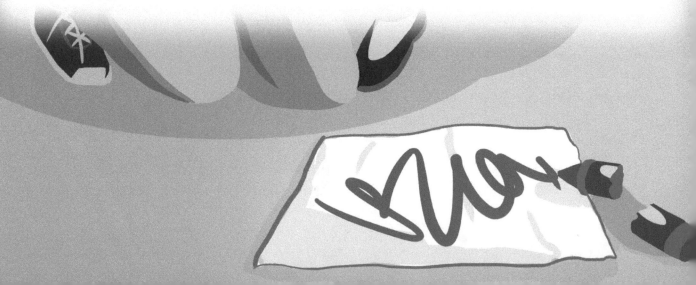

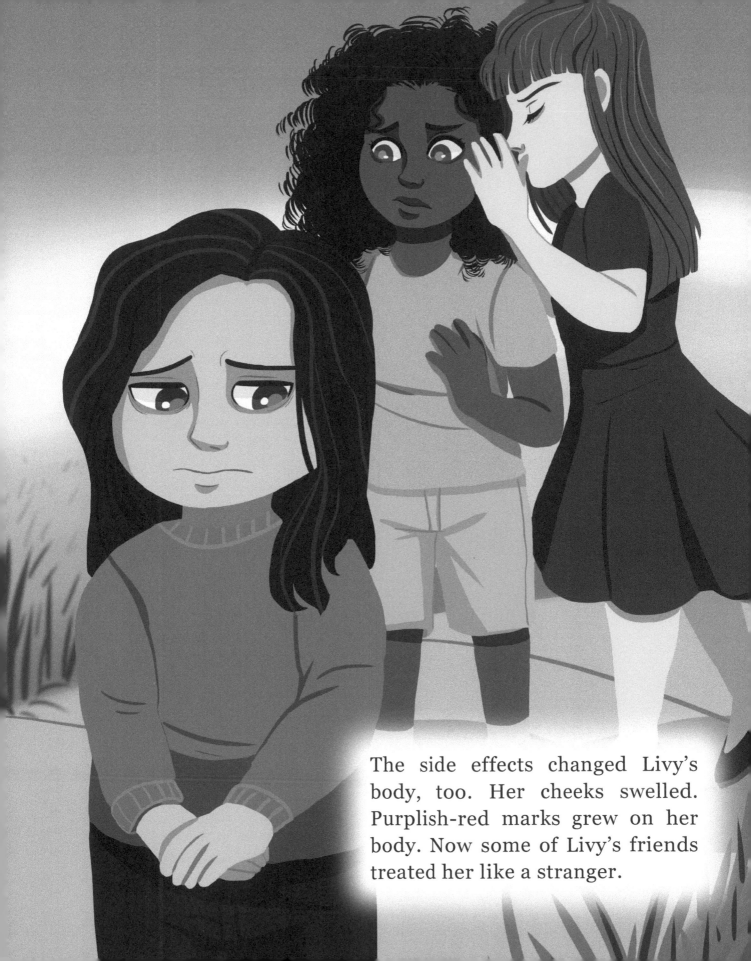

The side effects changed Livy's body, too. Her cheeks swelled. Purplish-red marks grew on her body. Now some of Livy's friends treated her like a stranger.

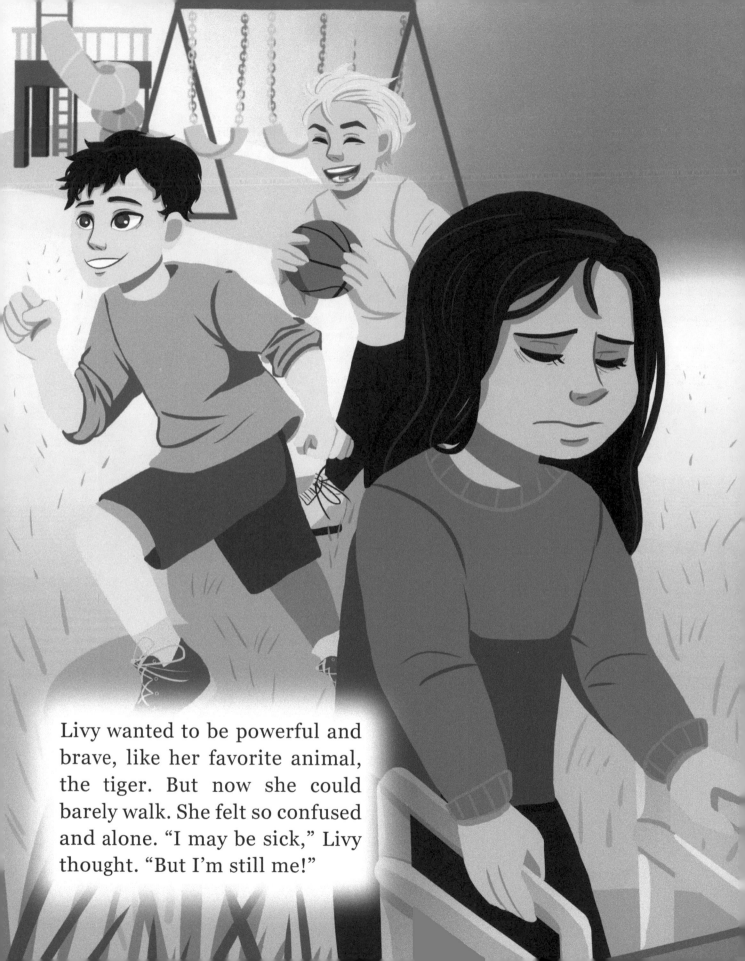

Livy wanted to be powerful and brave, like her favorite animal, the tiger. But now she could barely walk. She felt so confused and alone. "I may be sick," Livy thought. "But I'm still me!"

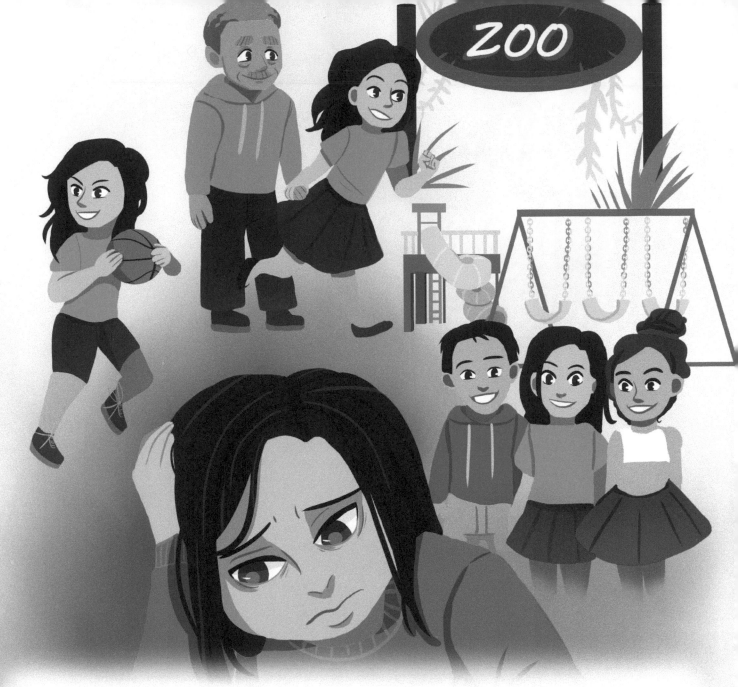

The medicine and the disease made her skin very sensitive to the sun. Livy was sad she now had to stay inside. She missed all the outdoor fun she used to enjoy and started to feel jealous. It was unfair she couldn't do all the things her friends got to do.

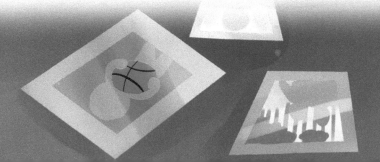

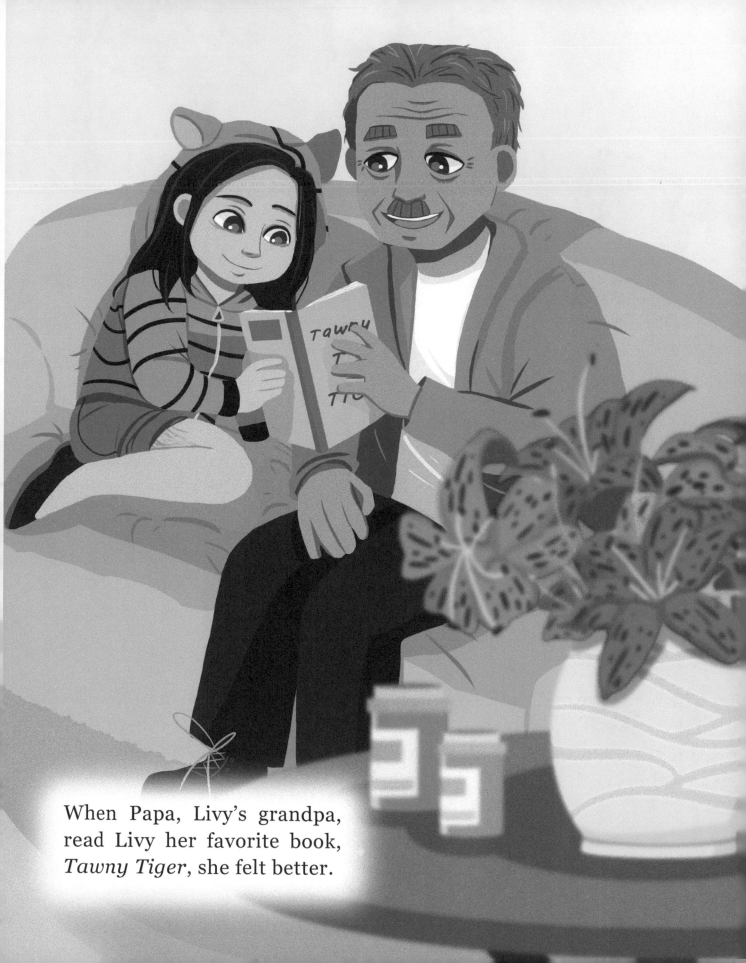

When Papa, Livy's grandpa, read Livy her favorite book, *Tawny Tiger*, she felt better.

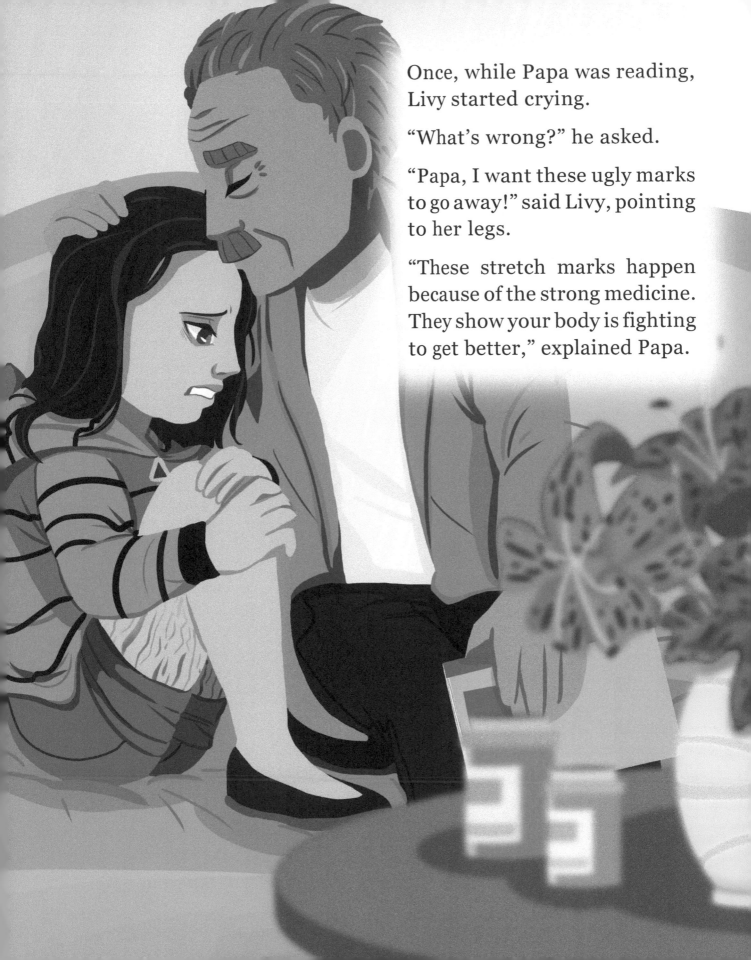

Once, while Papa was reading, Livy started crying.

"What's wrong?" he asked.

"Papa, I want these ugly marks to go away!" said Livy, pointing to her legs.

"These stretch marks happen because of the strong medicine. They show your body is fighting to get better," explained Papa.

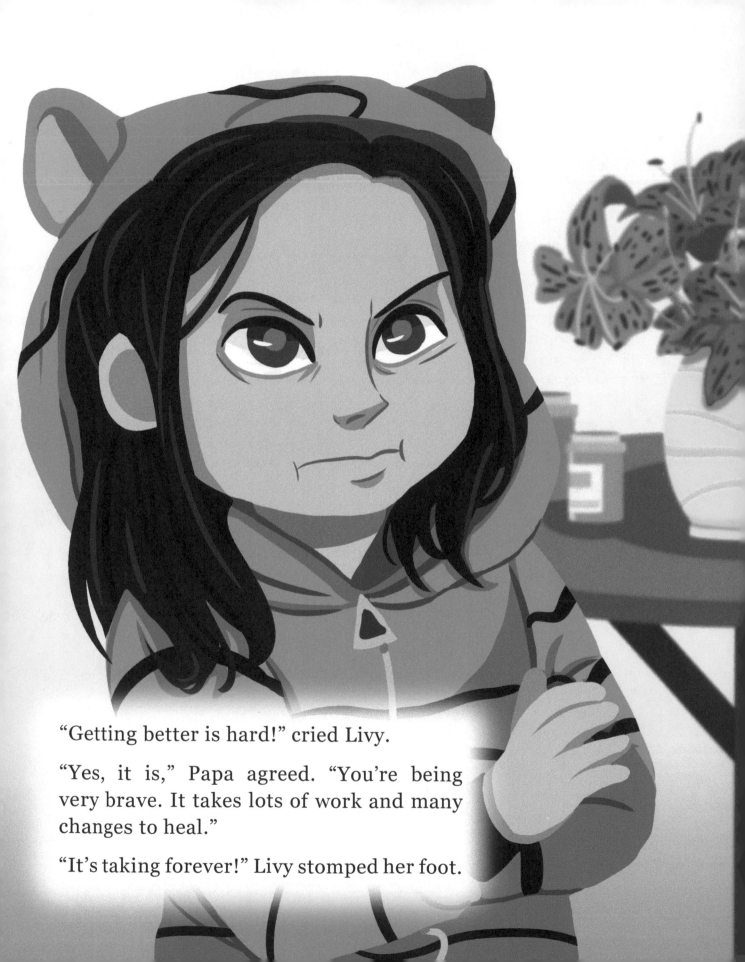

"Getting better is hard!" cried Livy.

"Yes, it is," Papa agreed. "You're being very brave. It takes lots of work and many changes to heal."

"It's taking forever!" Livy stomped her foot.

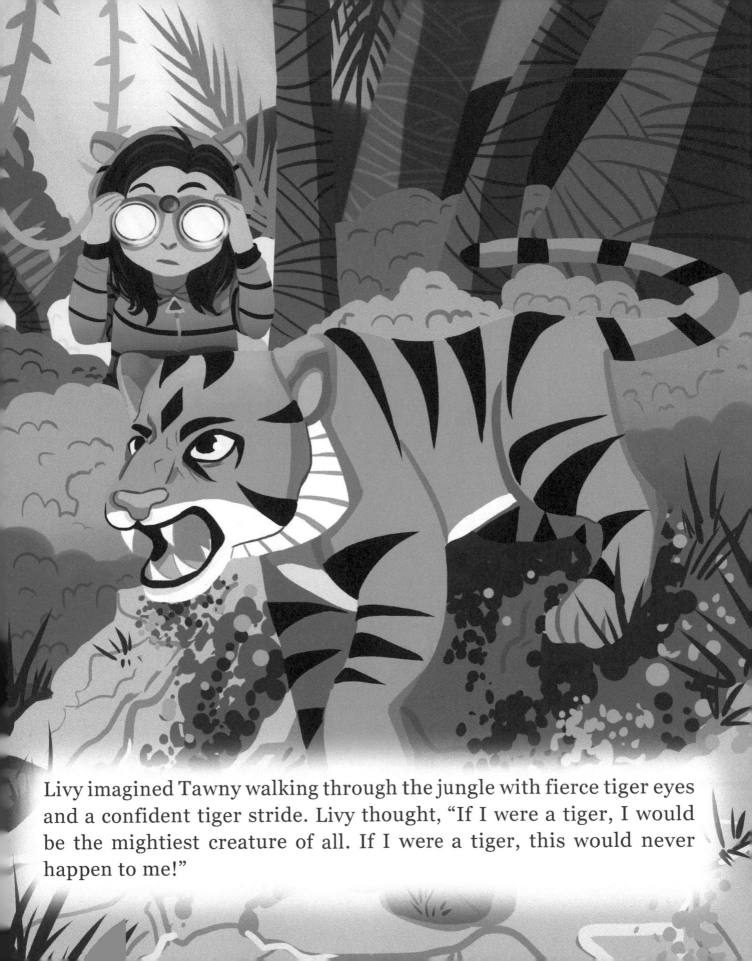

Livy imagined Tawny walking through the jungle with fierce tiger eyes and a confident tiger stride. Livy thought, "If I were a tiger, I would be the mightiest creature of all. If I were a tiger, this would never happen to me!"

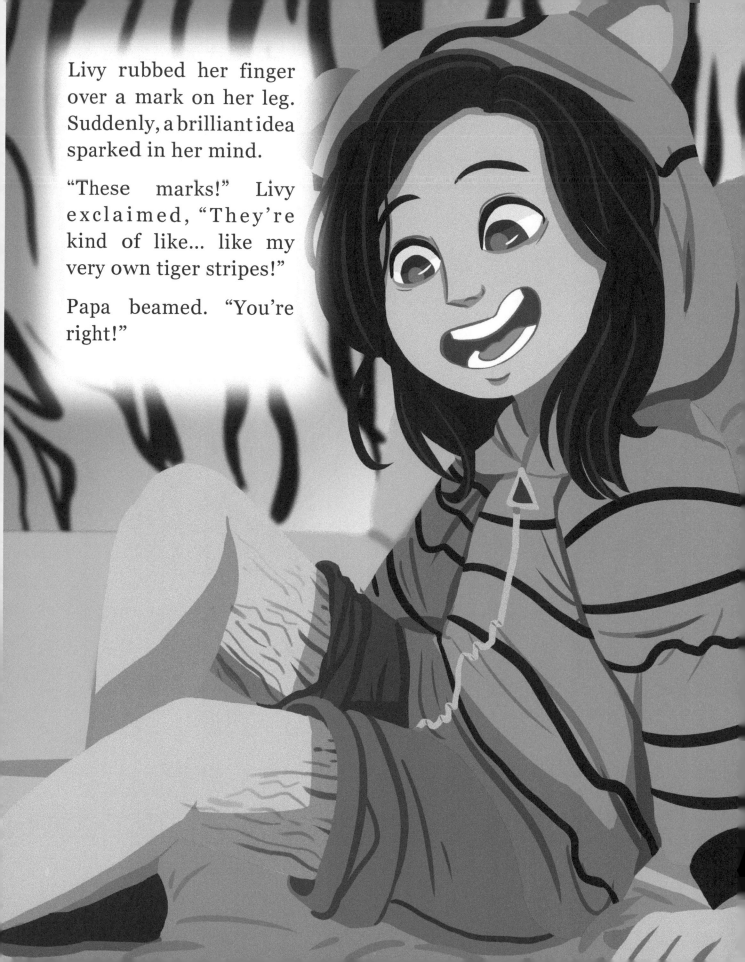

Livy rubbed her finger over a mark on her leg. Suddenly, a brilliant idea sparked in her mind.

"These marks!" Livy exclaimed, "They're kind of like... like my very own tiger stripes!"

Papa beamed. "You're right!"

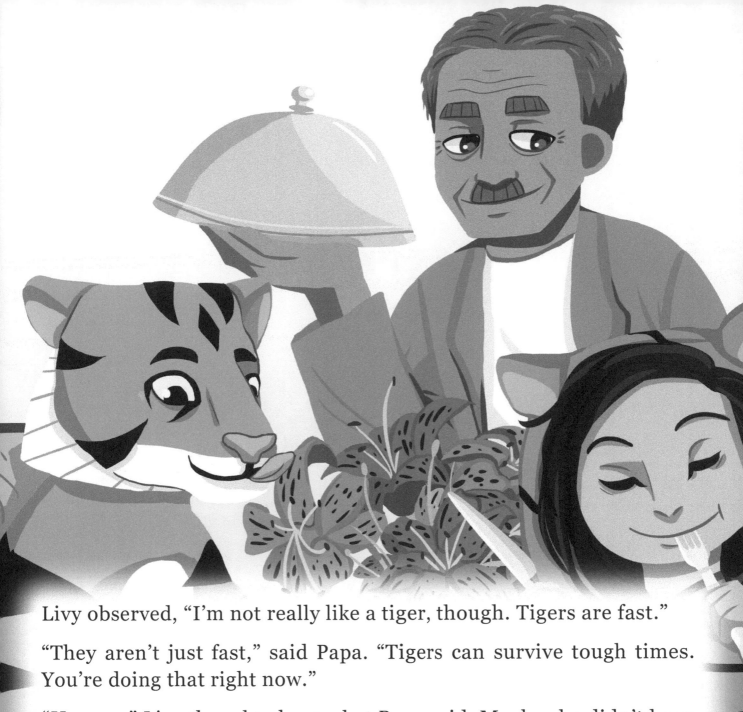

Livy observed, "I'm not really like a tiger, though. Tigers are fast."

"They aren't just fast," said Papa. "Tigers can survive tough times. You're doing that right now."

"Hmmm," Livy thought about what Papa said. Maybe she didn't have to be exactly like a tiger. After all, she was glad she didn't have to hunt for food.

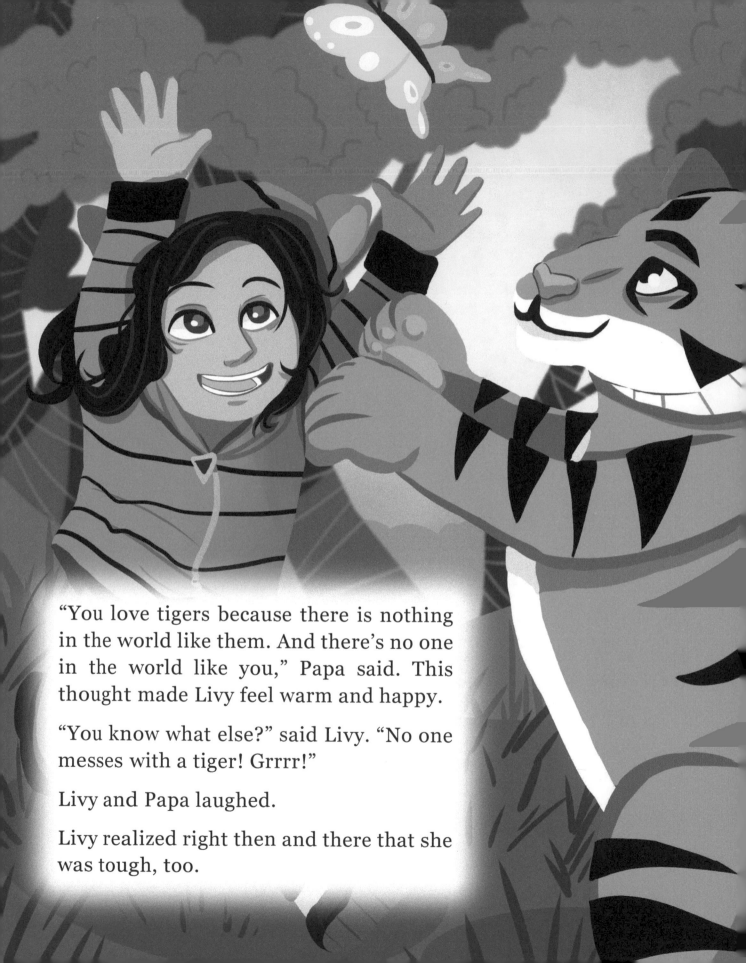

"You love tigers because there is nothing in the world like them. And there's no one in the world like you," Papa said. This thought made Livy feel warm and happy.

"You know what else?" said Livy. "No one messes with a tiger! Grrrr!"

Livy and Papa laughed.

Livy realized right then and there that she was tough, too.

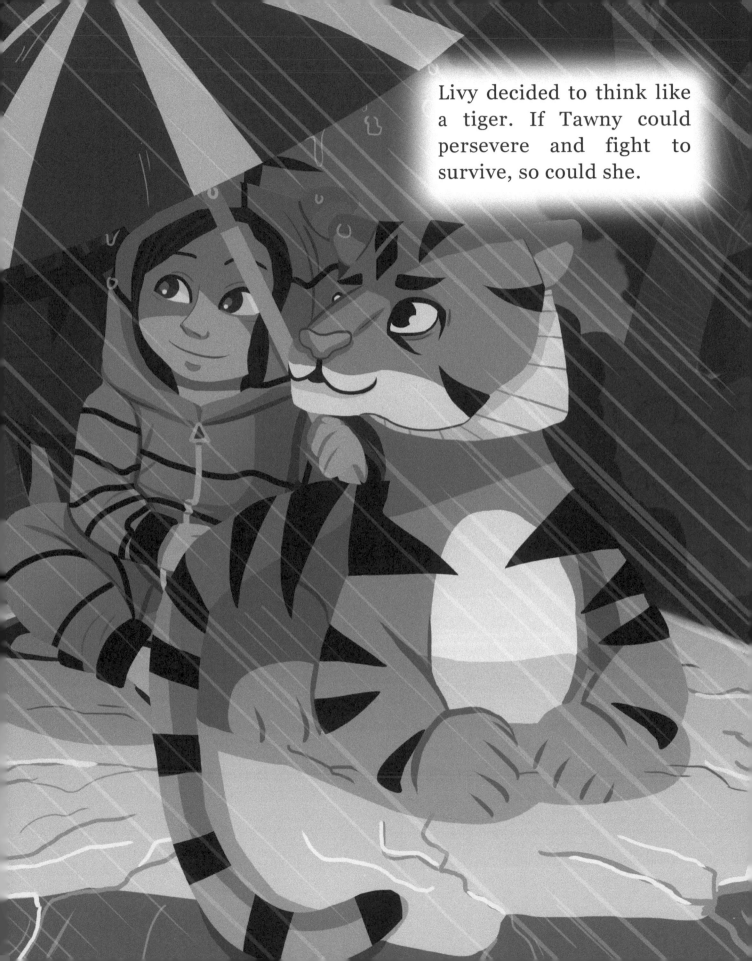

Livy decided to think like a tiger. If Tawny could persevere and fight to survive, so could she.

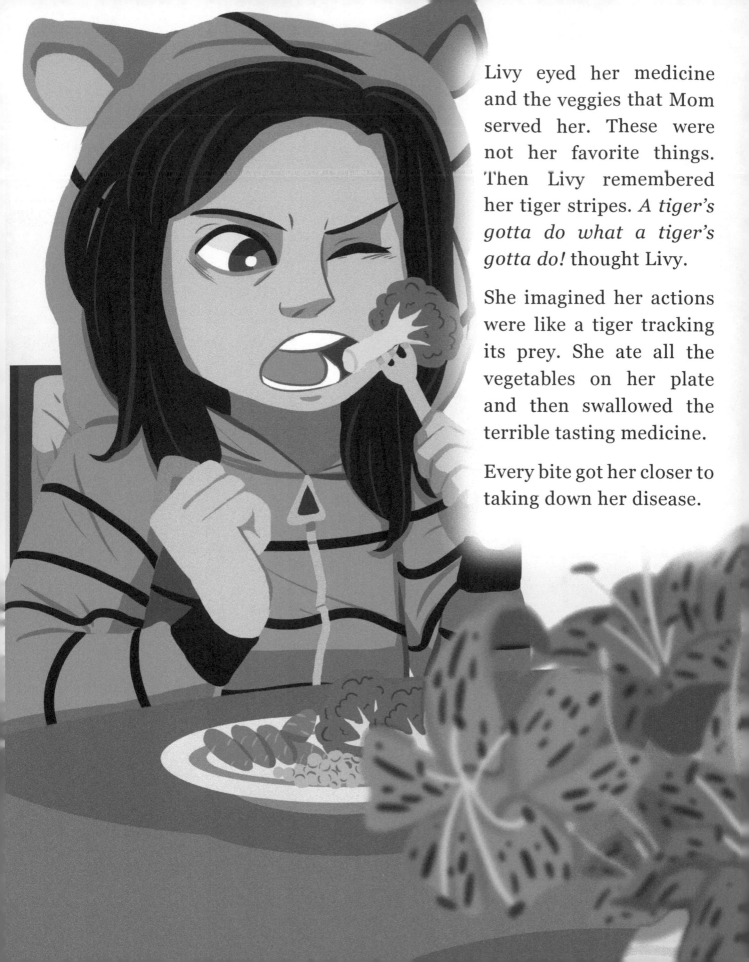

Livy eyed her medicine and the veggies that Mom served her. These were not her favorite things. Then Livy remembered her tiger stripes. *A tiger's gotta do what a tiger's gotta do!* thought Livy.

She imagined her actions were like a tiger tracking its prey. She ate all the vegetables on her plate and then swallowed the terrible tasting medicine.

Every bite got her closer to taking down her disease.

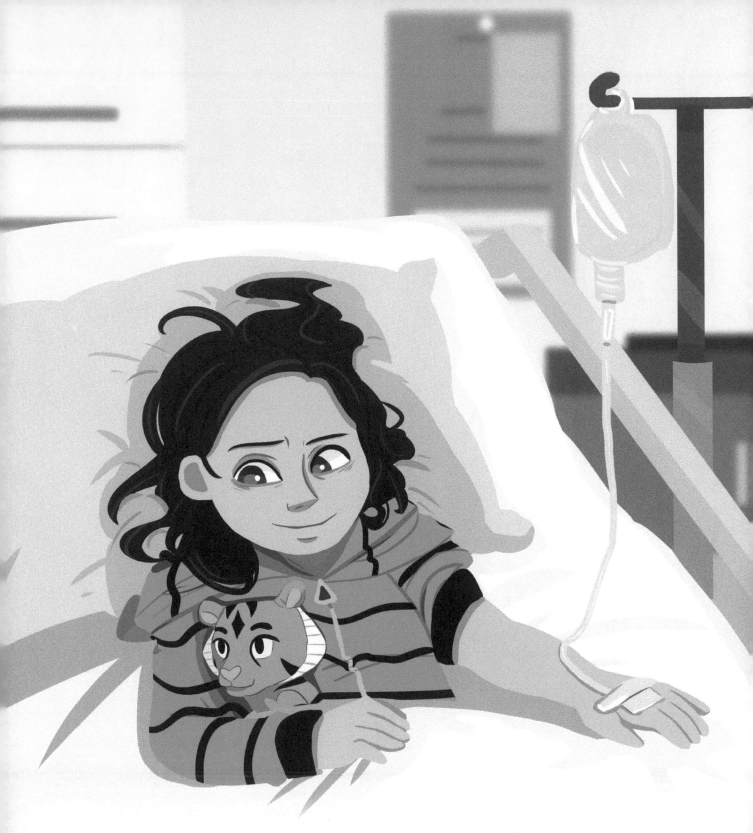

Thinking like a tiger made hard stuff like having an IV a little easier.
Just like a tiger, Livy patiently waited for her body to heal.

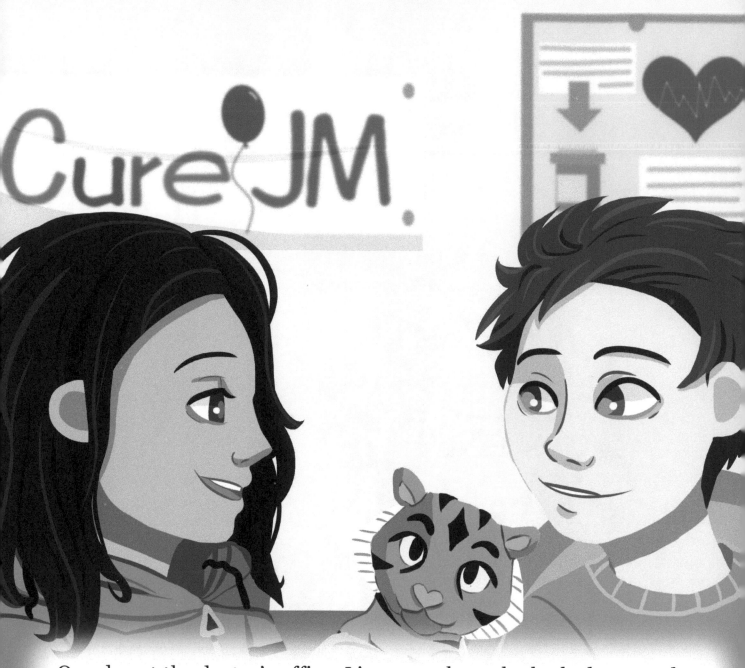

One day at the doctor's office, Livy saw a boy who looked very sad.

"Hi! My name is Livy and I'm getting a shot. Do you have to get a shot too?" she asked.

The boy nodded.

Livy looked in his worried eyes and said, "It's hard to get healthy. We have to be brave like tigers." They shared a smile.

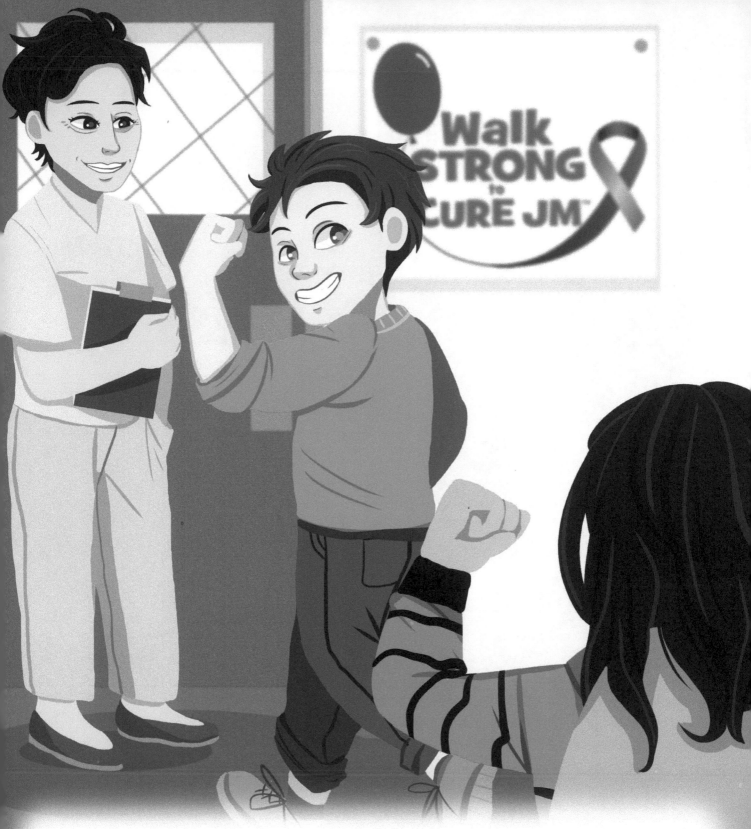

When the nurse called the boy for his shot, Livy waved and whispered, "Be brave, little tiger!"

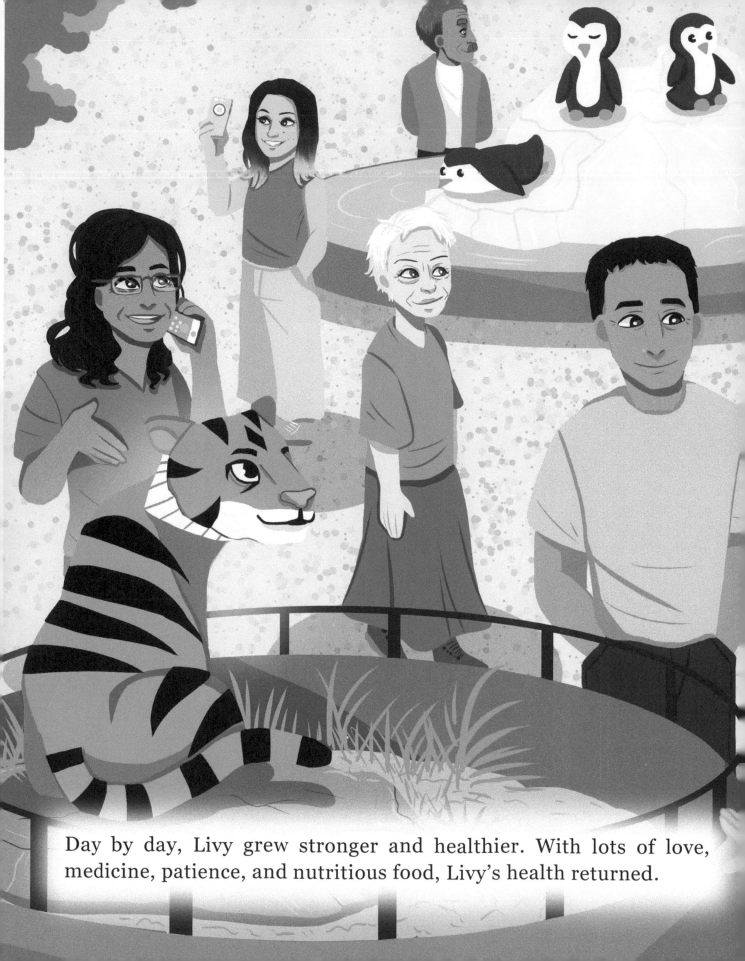

Day by day, Livy grew stronger and healthier. With lots of love, medicine, patience, and nutritious food, Livy's health returned.

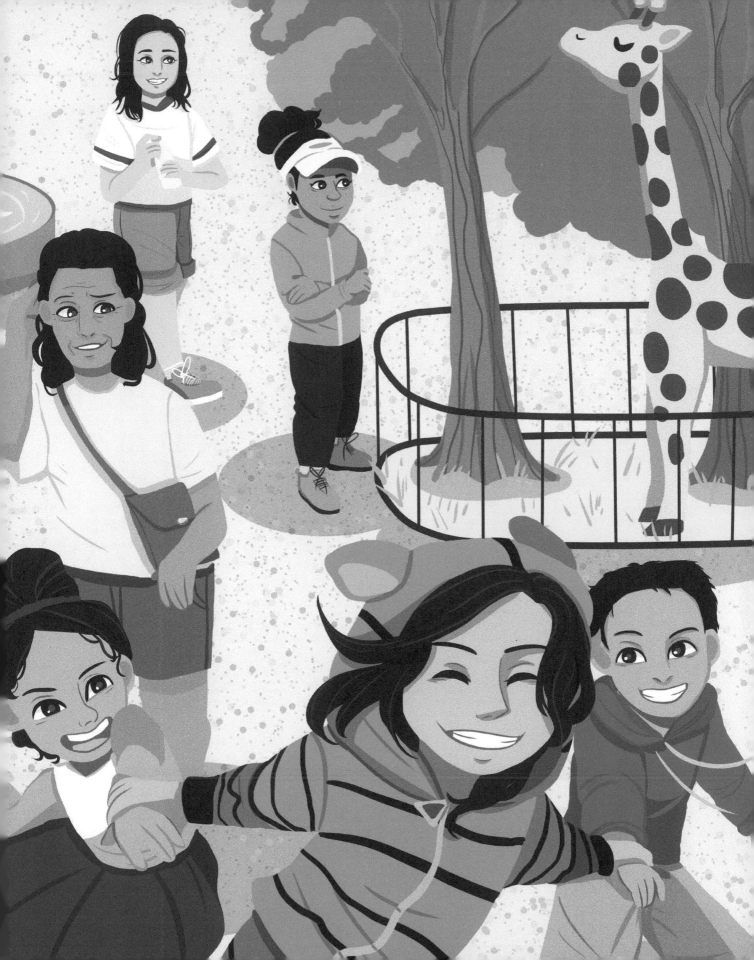

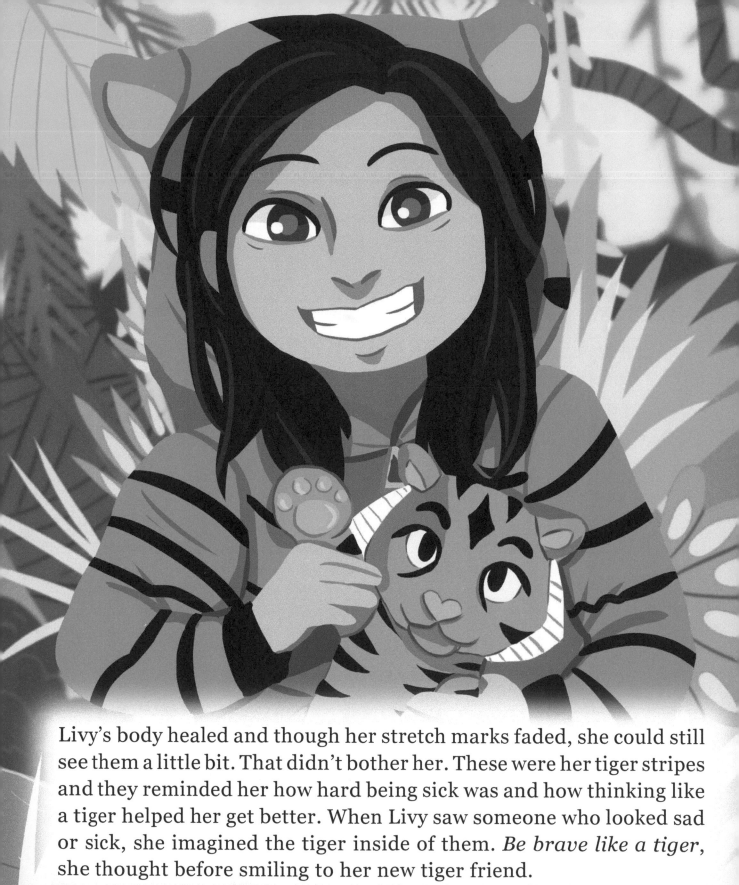

Livy's body healed and though her stretch marks faded, she could still see them a little bit. That didn't bother her. These were her tiger stripes and they reminded her how hard being sick was and how thinking like a tiger helped her get better. When Livy saw someone who looked sad or sick, she imagined the tiger inside of them. *Be brave like a tiger*, she thought before smiling to her new tiger friend.

About the Project

Thank you for supporting *Tiger Livy*. This book is inspired by coauthor Erin Garcia's niece, Livy, who was diagnosed with Juvenile Dermatomyositis (JDM or JM) at five years old. This rare disease causes a child's immune system to attack their own body. JM begins with muscle weakness and a rash. It can be mild or so severe that it is life-threatening.

Proceeds from this book will be donated to the Cure JM Foundation to help fund research to find a cure.

We all want and often expect health, but anyone who has been seriously ill or helped a loved one with a disease knows how sickness can take over a person's entire life. Just thinking like a tiger can't solve all our problems, but the mental and emotional sides of healing are important to learn about.

Healing takes compassion, education, patience, and support from loved ones. Reading also helps us see the world differently and is a brilliant way to grow and learn.

Even if you've never endured a serious illness, having empathy is crucial to helping those who are suffering. We hope that *Tiger Livy* encourages our readers to be kind and to find ways to make their communities a little brighter. Consider joining the Tiger Livy Project, where you can share your inspiration with others. Go to the @TigerLivyProject on Instagram or Facebook (with parent permission) or check out our webpage at tigerlivyproject.com.

P.S.- It's been a slow road to recovery, but with the help of many, Livy is in first grade and doing great!

For more information about JM or to connect with other JM families, go to CureJM.org. Or find @_lovin_liv to see what Livy is up to these days! You can even write a note to the real Livy at P.O. Box 319 Camarillo, CA 93011.

About the Authors and Illustrator

Erin Garcia is a public educator in the beautiful and robust Central Valley of California where she lives with her family. Garcia believes a person's health is both a personal and community effort. In her effort to walk the walk, she wrote a story to inspire people, connect communities, and generate donations to help find a cure for the heinous autoimmune disease JM. You can read about her latest projects at eringarciabooks.com.

Betsy Miller is the author of the picture book *Hip, Hop, Hooray for Brooklynn!* and the nonfiction books *The Parents' Guide to Perthes, The Parents' Guide to Clubfoot,* and *The Parents' Guide to Hip Dysplasia*. Miller joined this project to create a child-centered story that reflects the wonderful kids and families who bravely face children's health issues. Get to know her more at betsymillerbooks.weebly.com.

Ivreese Tong is an award-winning artist in the Central Valley of California and has practiced art for the past five years. Ms. Tong has experience with a plethora of art styles, subjects, and mediums. By illustrating this book, she hopes she can inspire others through her passion for art. Check out more of her beautiful work at ivreese.com.

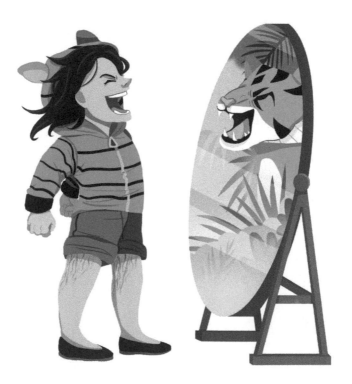

CPSIA information can be obtained
at www.ICGtesting.com
Printed in the USA
LVHW071801270921
698835LV00008BB/772

9 781733 856416